The Menopause Guide

Master the changes and stay youthful

By

Dr. Stacy Rose

I trust Stacy, always straight to the point. For me, it's more like a University lecture note.

Juliet Stones Co Founder, Women's Network.

Highly Informative and trusted for readers.

Vivian Vera

A Succinct but well presented for any woman out there.

Judith Potter. CEO, River Industry Ltd.

CONTENTS

INTRODUCTION

Around age 48, Joan recalls missing her period.
According to her mother, she entered menopause at age
50. She thus began to think, "Oh, we're getting started
now.

She also experienced some hot flashes and irregular
menstruation.
Her transition from perimenopause to menopause went
fairly smoothly. She found going through menopause to
be an isolating process. When women have their
periods, "there's more of a community experience," she
claims. Menopause is not a topic that women want to
discuss, as it is not a part of our culture or society. She
hadn't anticipated feeling better with her body as she
grew older. Joan believes that when she was in her 20s,
she had a very average body.

However, now that she has more time, she has
developed a great love for hiking, walking, and using her
body. She asserts that compared to when she was
younger, she is more athletic now.

She started doing a lot of things in her fifties. She runs a
gallery, paints, and launched her radio program when

she was 58. She has just recently—within the last five or ten years—had the time to complete the work she truly wanted to complete. At the age of 54, she experienced her first marriage. In her 20s and 30s, she claims she couldn't have envisioned this existence.

Joan claims to have very strong feelings about aging ladies.
I'm pretty pissed off about it, she says. Youth is a component of the societal perception of what makes a woman beautiful. Women are expected to seem young and beautiful regardless of their age in society. The stereotype, however, intensifies as we age. We will never, ever have true equality if we all want to be young. Menopause needs to change its image. It needs to be understood that it is a common experience shared by all women and that there is a full experience that follows that allows for a lot of freedom. We must embrace aging more positively and recognize all of its beneficial qualities.

She claims that despite spending time with young people, she doesn't strive to pass for one of them. She thinks she picks up knowledge from everyone and everything. She also constantly seeks out novel experiences. She asserts that staying active keeps one young.

Age 42, in a new relationship after many years as a single mom, physically fit, healthy, and active. Rose was in this.

The procedure to remove the breast mass from her was simple and surprisingly painless. She had no idea that the hormone-blocking medication (tamoxifen plus Zoladex) would cause issues.

Rose has always had compassion for women experiencing menopausal symptoms as a general practitioner who is interested in women's health.

But to be completely honest, she had always had the suspicion that some women were simply more likely than others to worry about their health. She was not one of those women. Rose, a feminist, didn't think her hormones defined or even significantly affected her. She says she was completely mistaken.

Overwhelming, draining, and unpredictable were the flushes. She alleges that she could not tolerate bedclothes or be touched in bed since she was nearly always overheated. Although she believes she knew some ladies who experienced such things as well, she was amazed that she could feel so heated without turning bright red or perspiring.

It was especially difficult to deal with the extreme fatigue.

She rested for 15-hour days - getting up was difficult for her. She said she lost all her inspiration and drive - just her youngsters and creatures made a big difference for her. My mindset plunged - despite a decent guess for her disease and a cherishing, steady family. She quit making arrangements for what's in store. Having been somebody who had consistently had a long-term plan (and accomplished it) this was all in all a change. She

felt disappointed for not adapting better - she'd
continuously serious areas of strength for testing times.
As such countless ladies do - She began
antidepressants.

They helped my state of mind a little - however, she had
no energy to get moving. She halted the chemical
treatment, against all clinical guidance and the requests
of my accomplice. She made a deal with God - simply
needing to see my youngsters through school.
In no less than about fourteen days, She felt improved -
more energy, less rest. Within 4 weeks, her
temperament moved along. In something like a year,
She was retraining to work, setting up another help, and
back to making her long-term plans! She was
anticipating the future once more.
Obviously, at 59 years of age, She has now gone
through menopause - which for me was less emotional.
She claims she misses estrogen - if it were restoratively
ok for her, she guarantees she would take it suddenly.
Her drive and libido are decreased - yet life is great.
She currently apologizes to any lady who she didn't treat
in a serious way as a GP. Estrogen is a phenomenal and
strong chemical, and its impacts ought to be regarded
immensely. Rose thinks we want to take a gander at
another way of life variable to truly uphold ladies through
menopause - diet, practice, care, and mental help.
To be positive, She thinks there are a few incredible
viewpoints to postmenopausal living! Life is smoother,
and more steady without the month-to-month cycle. God

has been benevolent to me, she asserts - She gets to see the delight of her youngsters developing into fit and kind grown-ups. She adds.

As a GP, she sees ladies confounded and shocked by the progressions menopause brings. We want more data and schooling about menopause - including the positive perspectives that things will improve.

The scene might have moved, however, when the seismic tremor settles nature dominates and the new biology secures itself. How about we embrace our chemicals when we have them yet not invest energy in grieving their misfortune? Life is more than the capacity to repeat - and postmenopausal ladies are a fundamental piece of our general public.

At long last, she says she is thankful for being a lady and every one of the encounters it brings. Chemicals might be a rollercoaster - however, the highs and lows have improved her life.

CHAPTER ONE: ABOUT MENOPAUSE

Menopause is a characteristic occasion for ladies.

Ahead of the pack up to menopause, your ovaries may not create an egg every month. This can prompt changes in the chemicals circling in your body. In particular, estrogen levels might be expanded and progesterone levels might be lower. After menopause, estrogen levels likewise fall impressively. Ladies are considered 'postmenopausal' one year after their last feminine period. Menopause happens at around age 50 however may happen prior because of chemotherapy, radiation therapy, or medical procedure.

What is menopause?

Menopause comprises three phases:

- The menopause progress (additionally called perimenopause). These are the years paving the way to the last feminine time frame and the year after the last feminine period. During this time, changes in your chemicals might prompt side effects, for example, hot flushes and changes in feminine draining examples. Night sweats (hot flushes happening around evening time) can cause rest aggravations and influence your mindset and fixation during the day. A few ladies are as yet ready to imagine during the menopause progress so you ought to keep on utilizing contraception until no less than a year after your last period on the off chance that you don't wish to become pregnant.

- Normal menopause is the unconstrained, extremely durable finish to feminine periods that isn't brought about by clinical treatment or medical procedures. It is affirmed by twelve continuous months of no feminine dying.

- Postmenopause is the time one year after your last menstrual bleeding and goes on until the end of your life.

HOW WILL MENOPAUSE AFFECT ME

Menopause unexpectedly influences each lady. Most ladies (around 85%) get a few hot flushes as well as night sweats, however, can deal with these without treatment. Around 20% of ladies have side effects that are irksome as well as drawn out and these ladies might think about treatment. The experience of menopause and side effects contrast in ladies from various ethnic gatherings, for instance, for a few Asian ladies, body and joint painfulness are the most problematic side effect.

Factors that may affect your menopause

- Your age at menopause. More youthful ladies who were not hoping to go through menopause might have more trouble than ladies at the typical age.

- Ladies who hope to have irksome menopausal side effects are bound to encounter problematic side effects when they go through menopause. In this way, a positive and informed way to deal with menopause might help.

- Numerous ladies are feeling better that they never again have periods and they feel relieved.

WHEN DOES MENOPAUSE BEGIN

Menopausal side effects (hot flashes, night sweats, feminine changes) as a rule start from around age 47 years. The last feminine time frame is as a rule about age 51 yet can fluctuate extensively. There is at present no dependable method for anticipating when you will encounter menopause and what your menopausal side effects will be like.

the point when menopause occurs before 40 years it is called 'untimely', and when it occurs before 45 years it is called 'early'. Menopause after age 45 years is viewed as ordinary and there could be no upper age cutoff to when it can start. In any case, most ladies have encountered menopause by age 55 years.

WHY DOES MENOPAUSE HAPPEN

The purposes behind menopause are not surely known. Right now, we imagine that menopause happens because the ovaries run out of eggs. This prompts changes in the chemicals created by the ovaries and the chemicals from the cerebrum that control the ovaries. In the long run, the ovaries quit delivering eggs and feminine periods stop forever. After menopause, the ovaries keep on creating estrogen at lower levels.

WHEN MENOPAUSE COMES EARLY

There are risks associated with early menopause:

- Loss of fruitfulness at a more youthful age.
- An expanded gamble of osteoporosis and break in ladies who don't take menopausal chemical treatment (MHT).

Early menopause is especially challenging for ladies who have not yet begun or finished their families.

CHAPTER TWO: HOW MENOPAUSE AFFECTS YOUR BRAIN

Menopause is a condition of regenerative senescence in the female. It starts in center life, including both neurological and endocrine maturing. It goes through various stages and is brought about by the decrease in female sex chemicals.

Menopause-related drops in capability might be the aftereffect of normal maturing of the endocrine hub or brought about by the expulsion of the ovaries or clinical treatment that forestalls ovarian endocrine capability.

Be that as it may, menopause is likewise a neurological change, as shown by numerous trademark side effects of menopause, particularly carelessness, rest unsettling influences, modified temperament, and hot glimmers. Ovarian and cerebrum well-being are thus inseparably connected in ladies.
As estrogen levels fall, changes happen in the morphology, number, and connections between nerve cells, their glucose digestion, and quality articulation. In female creature models, low estrogen has been

connected to the amassing of the strange protein amyloid-beta (Aβ), which is famous for shaping plaques inside cerebrum tissue, in individuals with Alzheimer's sickness (Promotion), however additionally some of the time in typical individuals.

ladies, this occurs in their 30s, and careful expulsion of the ovaries causes quick menopause, as do some disease medicines.) Those vacillations cause unpredictable periods and possibly a wide assortment of side effects, including hot glimmers, a sleeping disorder, temperament swings, inconvenient packing, and changes in sexual excitement. During this stage, known as perimenopause, which midpoints four years long (but can endure from a while to 10 years), Mosconi and partners saw that their female subjects encountered a deficiency of both dim matters (the synapses that interact data) and white matter (the filaments that interface those phones). Postmenopause, nonetheless, that misfortune halted, and now and again cerebrum volume expanded, however not to its premenopausal size. The analysts additionally distinguished comparing shifts in how the mind utilized energy, yet these didn't influence execution on a trial of memory, higher-request handling, and language. This proposes that the female cerebrum "goes through this interaction, and it recovers," says Jill M. Goldstein, a teacher of psychiatry and medication at Harvard Clinical School and pioneer and chief overseer of the Development Community on Sex Contrasts in Medication at Massachusetts General Medical clinic. "It adjusts to another typical."

Understanding what occurs in the mind around the hour of the menopause change could illuminate when and how specialists treat a given lady's side effects. Chemical treatment — whether estrogen alone or in blend with a progestogen — isn't normally recommended until postmenopause, and conveys gambles; then again, it can assist with treating hot flashes, bone issues, or unwanted urinary or vaginal changes for ladies under 60 (or who have started menopause inside the beyond 10 years), as per the North American Menopause Society. A few ladies who get chemical treatment could likewise acquire mental advantages, however, more proof is expected to recognize who ought to be dealt with. Randomized control preliminaries of postmenopausal ladies have attempted to evaluate whether chemical treatment diminished the gamble of Alzheimer's sickness or other mental degradations, yet these have returned blended results up until this point.

However, Mosconi and partners found that ladies in their review who had a specific hereditary gamble factor for Alzheimer's sickness started to foster amyloid plaques, which are connected to the illness, during perimenopause in their late 40s and mid-50s — sooner than previously suspected. Assuming that the mind changes essentially during perimenopause, that could end up being an urgent window during which to attempt to forestall Alzheimer's and other constant infections that frequently go with more established age. (Since chemical treatment isn't by and large recommended for perimenopausal ladies, clinical preliminaries on its potential mental advantages have not been finished for them.)

A few significant constant sicknesses, including Alzheimer's, seem to excessively burden ladies. As Goldstein and her partners noted in a January assessment segment in JAMA Psychiatry, more than 66% of those determined to have Alzheimer's are ladies (just to some degree since they live longer, and more established individuals are at more serious gamble). Ladies, as well, are at two times the gamble of fostering a significant burdensome problem, and they do as such pair with cardiovascular infection at two times the rate men do — a mix, the creators bring up, that expands their gamble of death from cardiovascular causes as much as fivefold. Coronary illness is likewise a gambling factor for Alzheimer's.

Sorting out why those well-being inconsistencies exist and what to do about them will expect analysts to consider sex and orientation explicitly as factors, which science has been delayed to do. Throughout recent years, for instance, scientists expecting to comprehend age-related mental degradation have commonly broken down information from people altogether, darkening contrasts between the genders to the extent that when deficiencies will generally show up and how to analyze them. "We want to ponder planning studies from the beginning in a manner that is pertinent for ladies and men," says Janine Austin Clayton, head of the Workplace of Exploration on Ladies' Wellbeing at the Public Foundations of Wellbeing. "Most people go through conceptual maturing, yet in particular ways," she says.

Another test is isolating the effects on well-being brought about by maturing versus those brought about by the hormonal changes that go with menopause. Preferably, you would look at countless ladies who are encountering them to ladies of a similar age who are not. Be that as it may, by their 50s, most ladies have reached perimenopause; by their 60s, practically all are postmenopausal. Mosconi and her associates represented this by contrasting ladies and age-matched men. In any case, as Stephanie Faubion, head of the Mayo Facility Community for Ladies' Wellbeing and clinical overseer of the NAMS, calls attention to, "Men's cerebrums will be unique concerning ladies."

The way that ladies can encounter huge cerebrum switches during menopause likewise brings up issues about how regularly this occurs and the degree to which it influences ladies' day-to-day routines, says Pauline Maki, a teacher of psychiatry, brain research, and obstetrics and gynecology at the College of Illinois at Chicago School of Medication. It's significant to note, she says, that ladies as often as possible report mental shortages around menopause, and that such side effects are normally brief. In any case, her work has shown that they are bound to lastingly affect low-pay ladies of variety — presumably, she says, since those ladies have higher paces of pressure, upset rest and that's what other psychological well-being loads "make the mind more powerless."

On the other hand, there are various conceivable preventive measures to safeguard mental well-being when the menopause change. Going without tobacco, being genuinely dynamic, eating a plant-rich eating regimen, decreasing pressure, and getting sufficient rest — are ways of supporting mind capability. Accordingly, it's a significant time for her to check in with her medical care supplier and examine her regenerative history and menopause status, every one of which can impact her illness hazard and therapy choices. Thus, suppliers of various types should be ready to focus on ladies all through their progress: "It's not simply in that frame of mind of gynecology," Faubion says, "and we need to quit considering it that way.

THREE WAYS MENOPAUSE AFFECTS YOUR BRAIN

1. Hormonal Changes neurotransmitter Production

Sex chemicals interface profoundly with mind synapses, including serotonin, GABA, glutamate, and dopamine.

Estrogen: influences emotions and neurotransmitter Production in numerous ways, including:

- Affecting serotonin levels and serotonin receptors.

- Changing endorphin levels, the "vibe great" synthetics.
- Adjust the pressure by affecting the arrival of stress synapses, like epinephrine and norepinephrine.

Estrogen is known to have a powerful serotonin-modulating effect by regulating the enzyme involved in its production (tryptophan hydroxylase), breakdown, and receptor sensitivity. The effectiveness of estrogen on serotonin availability lies on several factors, such as the amount of estrogen available.

Estrogen may also regulate stress by influencing the release of stress neurotransmitters, such as epinephrine and norepinephrine. It is also likely that hormone changes in the menopausal stage could impact the breakdown of stress neurotransmitters and serotonin.

Progesterone: While not talked about nearly as much as estrogen, progesterone also plays a crucial role in perimenopause and mood. Allopregnanolone, a downstream progesterone metabolite, has been said to modulate GABA (Gamma-aminobutyric acid) receptors resulting in anti-anxiety and antidepressant effects in clinical studies.

Progesterone has also been found to influence serotonin. This is through altering the expression of serotonin-related genes and proteins.

Some preliminary evidence indicates that progesterone is also neuroprotective in the brain, which could also impact one's tolerance to stress.

2. Temporary Memory & Cognitive Declines

Menopausal women can experience problems with learning and memory as estrogen levels dip. Estrogen has special nerves that play an essential part in our brains. These receptors are found within the limbic part of the brain (an area that controls mood and emotion). Presently, two receptors for estrogen in the limbic part of the brain have been identified, ER-alpha (ERalpha) and ER-beta (ERbeta). ERalpha regulates reproductive neuroendocrine behavior and function. ERbeta plays a role in nonreproductive behaviors, such as learning and memory, anxiety, and mood.

When these hormone levels dip, every system communicating with them, including your brain, marks these changes. So, it makes sense that when estrogen levels dips, as in menopause, cognition, and mental functioning can temporarily change due to all the different areas it controls in the brain. The good news is, this is usually not permanent, and rebalancing estrogen levels have been shown to modulate cognitive function.

3. The Structure of The Brain Changes

The ventral limbic and medial temporal lobe brain areas can be changed in menopause. These parts influence the consolidation of negative emotional information. This is possibly influenced by the presence of estrogen receptors in this area, as noted above. This impact on brain function may also cause mood changes and memory problems.

A new study used several types of brain imaging, magnetic resonance imaging (MRI), magnetic resonance spectroscopy to scan the brains of 161 women between the ages of 40 and 65. Some of the women were menopausal (one year without menstruation), some were transitioning to menopause ("perimenopause"), and a third group was postmenopausal

What Can Women Do to Maintain their Brain During Menopause?

Since most changes in the female cerebrum during menopause are impacted by hormonal movements, zeroing in on regular ways to deal with advanced hormonal equilibrium and mental capability is fundamental.

MOVEMENT

Expanded oxygenation and bloodstream from practice upgrade substantial help to all organ frameworks, including the cerebrum. Data are abundant on how exercise can further develop the mind and mental well-being, upgrade cerebrum development, and work with psychological facilities.

Summed up cerebrum impacts remember a lift for the number of veins and neurotransmitters, expanded mind volume, and diminished age-related mind decay. Restricted impacts incorporate developing new nerve cells and proteins to help these neurons make due and flourish. This further develops thinking and critical thinking abilities.

The best activity for one individual might contrast with another, as we are unique. All types of activity have support in the writing for further developing cerebrum wellbeing. Somewhere around 150 minutes of active work each week, however actually, it is possible that one needs to begin slowly and move gradually up to greater action.

Sustenance

An eating regimen wealthy in entire food sources, top-notch protein, omega-3-rich fats, and carbs (like the Mediterranean eating routine) has been displayed to usefully affect memory capability.

Remembering food sources rich in omega-3 unsaturated fats or enhancing with fish oil is particularly significant. Research exhibits relationships to fundamental unsaturated fats, mental health, and state of mind and conducts results.

Probiotic food varieties that help the stomach cerebrum pivot can likewise help. A few probiotics have been named "psychobiotic" which is a live creature that, when ingested in satisfactory sums, delivers a medical advantage in patients experiencing mental disease." These microbes have been found to deliver neuroactive substances, including GABA and serotonin, that can follow up on the stomach cerebrum hub.

Rest

Getting legitimate rest (roughly seven hours every evening) is basic for mental well-being. It assumes an urgent part in putting away and keeping up with memory and even aids clear the mind of the protein amyloid, one of the possible markers of likely Alzheimer's Sickness (Promotion) pathology.

Stress Decrease

Stress impacts the profound tone and can influence hormonal equilibrium. Studies have shown pressure decrease and loosening up strategies can free side effects from menopause and reduce strain, nervousness, and gloom while diminishing emotional episodes.

Menopause can make many changes in the mind connected with changes in chemicals, synapses, memory, cerebrum structure, and the stomach mind estrogen hub. Fortunately, this is normally brief, meanwhile, there are numerous ways of life, dietary, and supplemental help choices ladies can use to safeguard mental and mental capability.

CHAPTER THREE: HORMONE IMBALANCE. STEPS TO FIXING IT

A hormonal lopsidedness happens when you have excessively or excessively bit of at least one chemical. A wide term can address various chemical-related conditions.

Chemicals are strong signs. For a large number, having even somewhat excessively or excessively tad of them can make significant changes to your body and lead to specific circumstances that require treatment.

A few hormonal irregular characteristics can be brief while others are ongoing (long haul). What's more, a few hormonal lopsided characteristics require treatment so you can remain genuinely sound, while others may not influence your well-being but rather can adversely influence your satisfaction.

From the time ladies are conceived, their chemicals direct their craving, rest designs, how they answer pressure, drive, whether they will be cheerful or restless, and in the middle between. This happens when they're messed up.

The expression "Hormonal Imbalance" is tossed around a ton by well-being experts nowadays.

In any case, what does it mean? It sounds so nonexclusive and widely inclusive that most ladies are overpowered by the possibility of attempting to grasp this first piece of the riddle.

How would we try and know which chemicals are imbalanced, substantially less what side effects we ought to search for to sort out whether or not our chemicals are messed up?

At the point when most ladies under 40 hear "chemicals," it evokes pictures of menopause, hot glimmers, and emotional episodes.

The thing is, from the time ladies are conceived (well before menopause), chemicals are directing plenty of physical processes, similar to their hunger, rest designs, how they answer pressure, moxie, whether they are cheerful or restless, and in the middle between.

To this end, ladies of every age really should have a fundamental handle on how their chemicals work. In any case, we're looking about in obscurity for quite a long time, attempting to sort out a comprehension of what in blazes is happening in our bodies.

The chemicals that typically become imbalanced first are cortisol and insulin — "stress" and "glucose" chemicals, separately.

I call these the "alpha chemicals" since they downstream affect our thyroid, ovarian, and rest chemicals. As in, they disturb how thyroid chemicals, estrogen, progesterone, testosterone, and melatonin work in the body.

Alright, yet what's the significance here concerning side effects? Here is a portion of the principal indications of a chemical irregularity to pay special attention to:

- You experience difficulty nodding off or staying asleep for the entire evening.
- You battle to get up, indeed, even following seven to nine hours of rest.
- You want caffeine just to get going throughout the day.
- Do you want more caffeine or sugar?

around 10 a.m. and afterward again in the midafternoon to make all the difference for you.

Assuming you experience at least one of these side effects, you might have dysregulated cortisol, insulin, or both. All in all, what's a hormonally imbalanced young lady to do?

Make eating a careful practice

What you eat is similarly basically as significant as when and how you eat.

To keep up with what's known as adjusted glucose — and that implies you're keeping your glucose in a somewhat straight line as opposed to having huge spikes and plunges over the day — you ought to eat each three to four hours.

Kindly don't hold on until you're starving, have the shakes, feel like you'll hurl, or are weak. What's more, observe these guidelines at supper time. Slow it down, sweetheart.

Plunk down while eating, bite your food 20 to multiple times (I'm completely serious), and center around something positive while eating. At the point when you're worried, your stomach can only with significant effort assimilate the supplements you're consuming, so it doesn't make any difference how much broccoli you eat!

Scale back the cocktails

 Laying off the alcohol will be a distinct advantage.

A glass of liquor resembles consuming a small bunch of sweet treats, just through another conveyance strategy. It promptly hits your circulation system, sending your glucose levels on a thrill ride.

Liquor likewise raises estrogen levels, since it makes a ton of additional work for your liver, so it can't successfully detox estrogen, which is one of its fundamental positions. This estrogen abundance can set off heavier, longer periods, bosom agony, cerebral pains, and seething PMS.

See the association between what we eat and drink and our period issues?

Consider what caffeine is meaning to you

At the point when Joan converses with most ladies about caffeine, She ordinarily hears something as "I'll do anything you need me to, however, don't make me surrender espresso."

She comprehends that Life is nuts, and a large portion of us need to mainline caffeine just to squeeze by. This could be truly tricky, particularly assuming you experience uneasiness on the customary, feel like you can't get up toward the beginning of the day, have energy crashes in the day, or experience difficulty nodding off around evening time.

If you're not prepared to discard the joe, then see how you feel 30, 60, and 120 minutes after you've had an espresso. On the off chance that you're needing to tap out, slide into it with half decaf and half standard, supplant a cup a day with decaf, or trial with matcha.

Life is all out for so many of us nowadays, which is the reason I trust that you have a more clear image of what a chemical lopsidedness resembles and how to begin to switch it. Chemicals exist in a progressive system, so it's critical to take a "top-down" way to deal with resolving issues that emerge from a chemical irregularity.

Chemicals are additionally conversing with one another the entire day, so when you work on one chemical, the rest will begin to conform. That is the excellence of chemicals. They're cooperating to help you, consistently.

Diet and enhancements

Keeping a reasonable eating routine brimming with fundamental nutrients and minerals is vital to keeping up with generally speaking well-being. A solid eating routine incorporates lean and sound wellsprings of protein, solid fats, fiber, a lot of products of the soil, and insignificant sugar consumption. Concentrates on demonstrating the way that a few explicit supplements can assume a gigantic part in adjusting specific chemicals or focusing on unambiguous hormonal lopsided characteristics.

INOSITOL

Inositol might be an extraordinary choice for anybody battling with unpredictable periods, sporadic ovulation, and other fruitfulness-related hormonal uneven characteristics. Inositol's consequences for insulin flagging effects levels of chemicals like testosterone, insulin, and others. Inositol is found in food sources like organic products, beans, grains, and nuts. You can likewise take an inositol supplement to help cycle routineness.

Vitamin D

A suggested supplement for TTC, pregnancy, and general prosperity, vitamin D is viewed as a multifunctional chemical due to every one of its consequences for the body. Concentrates on showing that vitamin D supplementation might build chances of origination and increment AMH levels in certain ladies. We get vitamin D from sun openness, egg yolks, fish, and strengthened food sources.

Magnesium

Magnesium is a strong micronutrient that assumes a significant part in our sensory system, insulin discharge, and delivering and adjusting chemicals. Magnesium is tracked down in food varieties like dim mixed greens, seeds, vegetables, and avocados. Attempt Magnesium In addition to drinking blend for an extraordinary tasting method for supporting unwinding, calcium retention, and bone wellbeing.

Omega 3s

Omega 3 unsaturated fats are sound fats that can help the body in numerous ways. Our body utilizes these fats to forestall ADHD, and discouragement, and reduce aggravation. Studies have likewise shown that food sources containing omega-3 unsaturated fats might have the option to adjust chemicals and control the side effects of PCOS. Omega 3s must be eaten through enhancements and food varieties, like salmon, sardines, anchovies, pecans, seeds, and egg yolks.

Way of life changes

On top of focusing on a balanced eating regimen, numerous different pieces of our day-to-day schedules and ways of life can generally affect chemicals and chemical signs.

Stress decrease

While it's not exactly simple or easy, we could most likely benefit from bringing down our feelings of anxiety. High feelings of anxiety can significantly affect the body, including chemicals. Whether it's figuring out how to request help on a more regular basis, tracking down ways of remaining coordinated, or allowing yourself to express no to things all the more habitually, diminishing and overseeing everyday pressure can do incredible things for your well-being.

Focus on rest

Rest is a significant figure in hormonal equilibrium and guidelines. Chemical levels rise and fall over the day in light of your rest cycle, and if you're not getting sufficient tranquil rest around evening time, you could be seriously affecting your chemical motioning over the day.

Clinical Intervention

Clinical mediation might be important for a few hormonal uneven characteristics. Whether you have excessively or excessively bit of at least one chemical, your primary care physician might conclude that clinical treatment is important.

Hormone Replacement

There are oral drugs including estrogen and progesterone pills that might be endorsed by a specialist. You may likewise be recommended infusions for some chemical substitution. Talk with your medical care supplier about any various forms of feedback.

Medical procedure

While this isn't the main answer, generally speaking, there are times when medical procedures, radiation treatment, or a blend of clinical medications could be vital. This might be a choice if hormonal unevenness is brought about by cancer or another ailment. Talk with your medical services supplier about your circumstances.

Preventing Hormonal Imbalances

Intermittently there isn't a lot you can do to forestall hormonal uneven characters, nonetheless, keeping up with great by and large well-being is an extraordinary beginning. Consolidating solid propensities can assist with keeping your chemicals adjusted and assist you with precluding other possible causes if you do begin to see side effects of unevenness or endocrine problems. Solid propensities to keep up with or add to your routine incorporate eating a reasonable eating regimen, practicing consistently, getting a lot of rest, restricting liquor and tobacco, and tracking down ways of overseeing feelings of anxiety. It's additionally useful to stay away from EDCs, or endocrine-disturbing synthetic substances. These are synthetics that can affect the body because of their capacity to obstruct our regular chemicals. EDCs can hinder chemicals from working appropriately or can fool the body into believing they're chemicals. This might bring about an increment or abatement in certain chemicals. The most effective way to keep away from EDCs is to check your family items for normal EDCs, for example, phthalates, BPA, and others.

Assuming you're interested in your chemical levels, attempt an at-home testing unit or timetable a meeting with your PCP.

CHAPTER FOUR: IS BREAKFAST A HEALTHY THING

Breakfast is in many cases portrayed as the main meal of the day, however, is avoiding it truly negative to well-being? New studies suggest that it may not be as bad as some of us believe it to be.

Breakfast in a real sense signifies "to break the fast." It is the principal meal of the day after a stretch of not eating throughout the night.

Breakfast procured its title as the main meal of the day, harking back to the 1960s after American nutritionist Adelle Davis recommended that to stay in shape and stay away from corpulence, one ought to "have breakfast like a lord, lunch like a ruler, and supper like a homeless person."

However, a new investigation of 30,000 grown-ups found that 15% consistently skipped breakfast, and many trust it to be the main meal of the day. Breakfast gives the body significant supplements, to begin the day feeling stimulated and sustained. Many additionally accept that it can advance weight reduction.

However, is breakfast the main meal of the day?

Similarly, as with most things in nourishment, the response is perplexing. While some exploration recommends that skipping breakfast isn't destructive, another examination proposes in any case.

Eating standard meals and snacks, including breakfast, takes into account more open doors over the day to give the body the energy and supplements it requires to ideally work.

In any case, individuals can accommodate their supplements during different meals, breakfast may not be the most basic meal of the day.

Proof on the side of having breakfast

The greater part of the asserted advantages of having breakfast is fundamentally gotten from observational investigations, which can't demonstrate circumstances and logical results.

For instance, one 2021 deliberate survey of 14 observational examinations found that the individuals who have breakfast seven times each week have a diminished gamble for:

heart disease
diabetes
obesity
high blood pressure
stroke
abdominal obesity
cardiovascular-related death
elevated low-density lipoprotein (LDL) cholesterol.

Are people who eat breakfast healthier?

As per one 2018 observational review, the people who now and again have breakfast frequently focus harder on their general supplement admission, routinely partake in active work, and enough oversee pressure.

Alternately, the individuals who skip breakfast will more often than not have an unhealthier way of life propensities like regular smoking and drinking. They additionally will generally consume fewer calories higher in fat, cholesterol, and calories than routine breakfast eaters.

These discoveries recommend that way of life propensities might add to the general well-being status of breakfast eaters, not having breakfast.

Would it be advisable for you to have breakfast?

Since breakfast offers us the chance to fuel our body with supplements, it is a significant dinner. Be that as it may, as per ongoing investigations, it may not be the main dinner of the day.

Having breakfast and paying attention to your appetite signals is vital if you awaken hungry in the first part of the day. In any case, on the off chance that you get going and skip breakfast one day, there is a compelling reason to feel regretful.

Assuming you routinely skip breakfast, it is essential to guarantee you are enhancing your supplement admission at different dinners.

Certain gatherings, for example, wellness experts or competitors who train promptly in the first part of the day, may likewise feel improved in the wake of having breakfast.

What would it be advisable for you to have for breakfast?
On the off chance that you appreciate breakfast, start your day with nutritious food varieties.

Some healthy breakfast foods include:

eggs
oatmeal
Greek yogurt
berries
whole-grain toast
chia seeds
cottage cheese
avocado
nuts.

Here are five common health benefits of eating breakfast:

May safeguard your heart
As indicated by a new report, the individuals who didn't eat a morning dinner were bound to secure coronary illness more than the people who did.
As per research, individuals who skip breakfast put on weight, which can prompt diabetes, elevated cholesterol, and pulse, and these can build your gamble of coronary illness.
The specific clarification is obscure, however, breakfast captains are remembered to indulge in different feasts and nibble exorbitantly over the day.

Could bring down your gamble of type II diabetes
An early breakfast might assist you with keeping away from blood glucose changes, which can add to diabetes. Concentrates on a show that individuals more youthful than 65 years who skipped breakfast even a couple of times every week were 28% more bound to procure diabetes than the people who ate it consistently.

Great for memory
Breakfast might further develop memory, focus, the speed with which data is handled, thinking, imagination, learning, and talking gifts in the two grown-ups and youngsters as per research.
Researchers at the College of Milan in Italy broke down examinations and found proof that such advantages might be because of the consistent glucose levels given by a morning feast.

Holds your weight down
Even though reviews have associated having breakfast with a lower chance of corpulence, specialists demonstrated that those reviews are simply observational, and it can't be laid out that dinner forestalls weight gain.
Randomized controlled preliminaries give more dependable proof. As per research distributed in the Stoutness diary, overweight grown-ups who were eating fewer carbs and had a greater number of calories for breakfast than supper lost more weight than the people who ate bigger night dinners.

Better state of mind

A solid breakfast can further develop a mindset.

As per research, following a night's rest, eating toward the beginning of the day will renew your mind's glucose stores.

At the point when they aren't occupied by hunger sensations, the vast majority are probably going to be more joyful and less irritable.

Why is breakfast the main dinner of the day?

Breakfast is one of the main dinners of the day (for the most part). Breakfast eaters by and large have better weight control plans, polishing off additional organic products, vegetables, milk, and entire grains than non-breakfast eaters.

Breakfast unmistakably affects you more than some other dinner because the time between night and the following morning's feast is the longest your body does without sustenance. Eating within something like two hours of waking can influence how you process glucose over the day.

Breakfast is an imperative feast if you have any desire to keep up with your dynamic way of life. Essentially ensure you get your morning calories from an even feast. Making time to eat something nutritious toward the beginning of your day can altogether affect your general prosperity.

Having a sound breakfast is useful to your drawn-out wellbeing. It can assist with lessening weight, hypertension, the gamble of coronary illness, and diabetes.

CHAPTER FIVE: IS KETOGENIC ROUTE HELPFUL FOR MENOPAUSE

Certain individuals find that making diet and way of life changes assists with their menopause side effects. In any case, there is presently no proof that the keto diet, specifically, is advantageous.

The ketogenic or keto diet places the body into a condition of ketosis. This implies the body involves fat for energy, transforming it into ketones. It then utilizes these ketones rather than sugar.

To prompt ketosis, an individual needs to confine starch consumption and supplant it with fat. The keto diet normally comprises:

55-60% fats
30-35% protein
5-10% starches

The specific food sources an individual eats in the eating routine can differ. They can consume a lot of organic products, vegetables, and sound fats while in ketosis, yet eating bunches of red meat and soaked fat is similarly conceivable.

The keto diet might assist with arriving at a moderate weight, yet its effect on other menopause side effects is less clear.
Certain individuals experience weight gain during menopause, which might be a consequence of changes in chemical levels and more slow digestion.

There is no examination on whether the keto diet is a powerful method for keeping a solid load during menopause. In any case, an enormous 2017 investigation of almost 89,000 females matured 49-81 years contrasted four eating regimens with perceiving how well they functioned.

- a low-fat diet
- a low carbohydrate diet
- a Mediterranean-style diet
- a diet consistent with the United States Department of Agriculture's Dietary Guidelines for Americans

The specialists found that individuals who followed a low-carb diet had a lower chance of postmenopausal weight gain than other eating routines.

Be that as it may, in this review, the low-carb diet restricted sugars to 163 grams (g) each day. The keto diet is significantly more prohibitive than this, restricting sugars to under 50 g.
Individuals can encounter an expansion in hunger or food desires during perimenopause and menopause. Some examination recommends that the keto diet might diminish hunger, which might assist with these side effects.

For instance, a recent report including 55 female and 40 male members with weight took a gander at the keto diet and changes in hunger.

Specialists found that following the keto diet for quite some time expanded levels of the hunger-managing chemical glucagon-like peptide 1 in the female members. Strangely, the levels of this chemical diminished in the male members.

Be that as it may, the review didn't explicitly check out a hunger decrease during menopause. The members' ages went from 18-65, thus incorporating a combination of pre-and postmenopausal females.
There is right now no exploration on whether the keto diet helps or impedes the equilibrium of conceptive

chemicals during menopause, so the impacts on declining estrogen and progesterone levels are obscure.

Could keto free you once again from menopause?

No — no eating regimen, supplement, or drug can stop or oppose menopause. A characteristic stage in life happens when the body quits making as much estrogen and progesterone.

Notwithstanding, chemical treatment can supplant the chemicals an individual is losing, which can mitigate side effects.

Keto secondary effects

The keto diet can cause secondary effects, particularly when an individual initially beginnings the eating regimen. Many individuals experience "keto influenza," an assortment of side effects that emerge as the body enters ketosis. These can include:

headache
irritability
weakness
dehydration
dizziness
muscle soreness

Following a keto diet can likewise make it more testing to consume enough specific supplements. For instance, one investigation discovered that individuals who follow a keto diet consume less fiber.

Individuals might eat less leafy foods trying to stay away from sugars, meaning they get fewer nutrients, minerals, and prebiotics. Prebiotic fiber takes care of the useful microbes in the stomach.

A method for balancing this is to zero in on proceeding to eat a lot of fiber and new produce while following the keto diet.

Five Likely Gamble Of The Keto Diet

1. May prompt the keto influenza

Carb consumption on the keto diet is regularly restricted to less than 50 grams each day, which can come as a shock to your body

As your body drains its carb stores and changes to involving ketones and fat for fuel toward the beginning of this eating design, you might encounter influenza-like side effects.

These incorporate cerebral pains, wooziness, exhaustion, sickness, and clogging — due to some extent to parchedness and electrolyte-lopsided characteristics that occur as your body acclimates to ketosis

While the vast majority who experience keto influenza feel quite a bit improved within half a month, it's critical to screen these side effects all through the eating routine, remain hydrated, and eat food varieties wealthy in sodium, potassium, and different electrolytes.

 2. May pressure your kidneys

High-fat creature food sources, like eggs, meat, and cheddar, are staples of the keto diet since they don't contain carbs. On the off chance that you eat a great deal of these food varieties, you might have a higher gamble of kidney stones.

That is because a high admission of creature food sources can make your blood and pee more acidic, prompting expanded discharge of calcium in your pee. A few examinations likewise propose that the keto diet decreases how much citrate that is delivered in your pee. Considering that citrate can tie to calcium and forestall the arrangement of kidney stones, diminished degrees of it might likewise raise your gamble of creating them.

Moreover, individuals with persistent kidney sickness (CKD) ought to keep away from keto, as debilitated kidneys might not be able to eliminate the corrosive development in your blood that outcomes from these creature food sources. This can prompt a condition of acidosis, which can demolish the movement of CKD.

Additionally, lower protein abstains from food are frequently suggested for people with CKD, while the keto diet is moderate to high in protein.

 3. May cause stomach-related issues and changes in stomach microscopic organisms

Since the keto diet limits carbs, it tends to be hard to meet your everyday fiber needs.

Probably the most extravagant wellsprings of fiber, for example, high-carb organic products, boring vegetables, entire grains, and beans, are wiped out on the eating routine since they give such a large number of carbs.

Thus, the keto diet can prompt stomach-related inconvenience and stoppage.

A 10-year concentrate on youngsters with epilepsy on the ketogenic diet tracked down that 65% detailed clogging as a typical secondary effect.
Likewise, fiber takes care of the advantageous microbes in your stomach. Having a sound stomach might assist with supporting invulnerability, working on psychological well-being, and declining irritation.

A low-carb diet that is deficient in fiber, for example, keto, may adversely influence your stomach microbes — albeit flow research on this subject is blended

Some keto-accommodating food varieties that are high in fiber incorporate flax seeds, chia seeds, coconut, broccoli, cauliflower, and salad greens.

4. May prompt supplement inadequacies

Since the keto diet limits a few food sources, particularly supplements thick natural products, entire grains, and vegetables, it might neglect to give suggested measures of nutrients and minerals.

Specifically, a few investigations recommend that the keto diet doesn't give sufficient calcium, vitamin D, magnesium, and phosphorus.

A review that assessed the supplement structure of normal weight control plans uncovered that exceptionally low-carb eating designs like Atkins, which is like keto, gave adequate sums to just 12 of the 27 nutrients and minerals your body needs to get from food.

5. May cause perilously low glucose

Low-carb eats less like keto have been displayed to assist with overseeing glucose levels in individuals with diabetes.
Specifically, a few investigations propose that keto may assist with diminishing degrees of hemoglobin A1c, a proportion of normal glucose levels

Notwithstanding, people with type 1 diabetes might be at a high gamble of additional episodes of low glucose (hypoglycemia), which is set apart by disarray, flimsiness, weakness, and perspiring. Hypoglycemia can prompt unconsciousness and demise if not treated.

A concentration in 11 grown-ups with type 1 diabetes who followed a ketogenic diet for north of 2 years found that the middle number of low glucose occasions was near 1 every day.

People with type 1 diabetes normally experience low glucose on the off chance that they are taking an excess of insulin and not consuming enough carbs. Consequently, a low-carb keto diet might expand the gamble.

Hypothetically, this could likewise happen to people with type 2 diabetes who are taking insulin meds.

CHAPTER SIX: WHAT IS DETOXING

Nowadays, the word detoxification can be heard universally and is frequently utilized nonchalantly also. Be that as it may, comprehending its genuine embodiment, what it means, and how its true capacity can be bridled can improve things greatly.

Anyway, what's the significance here? detoxification is restorative and alludes to the normal expulsion of poisons from the body. On an everyday premise the liver, kidneys, digestion tracts lymphatic frameworks are accomplishing this turnout ceaselessly for us. Why is there a need to have an extra detoxification program for the body?

We are presented with countless synthetic compounds - be it in our food supply, the air we inhale, day to day we use of beauty care products, and other substance specialists in cleaning. A portion of these are exceptionally hurtful and can cause likely harm. To create the liver and kidney more productive we can take on a few sound practices, which thusly help to flush the poisons out.

There are different detox slims down going from absolute starvation diets to juice diets, to food adjustment approaches, and those that frequently include the utilization of intestinal medicines, diuretics, nutrients, minerals, and additionally 'purging food varieties". These all subject the body to unjustifiable pressure and turn out just for the present.

Detox diets may seriously restrict energy and supplement admission, presenting different dangers to

your well-being. A few gatherings ought to never detox and eats less.
However, there is no clinical examination that can uphold this methodology.

Detoxification ought to be a way of life change where the spotlight is more on eating clean food. It brings about purifying of the body, feeding and re-energizing it. One ought to initially zero in on diminishing the poison burden to the body and then eating such food sources, which can give sound supplements that will help in refueling the body.

The center ought to be to detox all parts of life. These poisons are generally the justification behind slowed-down weight reduction notwithstanding exercise and the right eating regimen. In this way, taking on the right program can support one's well-being and help in weight reduction. It will likewise cause one to feel more joyful and better from the inside.

Detoxification, frequently alluded to as detox, is a characteristic physiological cycle that happens in the body to dispense with or kill unsafe substances. It is the cycle by which the body takes out or changes poisons and side-effects to keep up with generally speaking well-being and prosperity.

The body has its detoxification instruments basically by organs like the liver, kidneys, lungs, skin, and digestion tracts. These organs cooperate to distinguish and dispose of poisons, metabolic side effects, and other destructive substances from the body.

Detoxification can likewise allude to explicit practices or projects pointed toward supporting and upgrading the body's regular detox processes. These projects normally include dietary changes, fasting, homegrown supplements, explicit conventions, or treatments that cause to purify the group of poisons and work on general well-being. Notwithstanding, it's vital to take note that the adequacy and logical proof behind such detox projects can change altogether.

It's worth focusing on that the human body is by and large exceptional to normally detoxify itself. The liver, specifically, assumes a critical part in sifting and handling poisons, while the kidneys assist with taking out side effects through pee. Driving a solid way of life, including a fair eating regimen, normal activity, legitimate hydration, and adequate rest, can uphold the body's regular detoxification processes.

If you have worries about detoxification or wish to leave on a detox program, it is prescribed to talk with a medical service proficient or enlisted dietitian who can give customized counsel in light of your singular necessities and well-being status.

SHOULD I DETOXIFY ?

Deciding whether you want to detoxify or on the other hand if your body needs help for its regular detoxification processes is a complicated matter. While certain people might profit from explicit detox projects or mediations, it's critical to move toward the idea of detoxification with alert and counsel medical care proficient for customized direction. Here are a few general signs that might propose the requirement for detoxification support:

1. Steady Exhaustion: If you continually feel tired and need energy notwithstanding sufficient rest, it very well may be an indication that your body's detoxification frameworks are overpowered or imbalanced.

2. Stomach-related Issues: Regular bulging, gas, stoppage, looseness of the bowels, or other gastrointestinal issues might show a gathering of poisons or impeded stomach-related capability.

3. Skin Issues: Skin conditions like skin break out, dermatitis, or rashes can at times be an impression of fundamental poisons or irregular characteristics in the body.

4. Weight Gain: Trouble getting more fit or unexplained weight gain, particularly around the stomach region, might be related to poison development or metabolic interruptions.

5. Mind Haze: Encountering mental fogginess, trouble concentrating, or unfortunate memory could show a requirement for detoxification support.

6. Substance Openness: If you have been presented with elevated degrees of ecological poisons, contaminations, or synthetic compounds, for example, through your occupation or living climate, supporting your body's detoxification pathways might be valuable.

It's essential to take note that these signs and side effects are not elite to poison gathering, and they can have different causes. Furthermore, the idea of detoxification programs or purges that case to "flush out" poisons isn't all around upheld by logical proof.

If you have worries about your well-being or suspect a requirement for detoxification, it is prescribed to talk with medical care proficiently. They can evaluate what is happening, perform pertinent tests if important, and give fitting directions and suggestions customized to your singular requirements.

IS DETOX GOOD FOR MENOPAUSE

Detoxification practices or projects are not innately designated explicitly for menopause, nor are they demonstrated to lighten menopausal side effects straightforwardly. Menopause is a characteristic natural progress in a lady's life when the ovaries stop delivering eggs and chemical levels vacillate, prompting different physical and close-to-home changes.

While some detoxification procedures might offer specific advantages for ladies going through menopause, it is crucial to approach them with alertness and talk with medical care proficient before making any critical dietary or way of life changes. Here are some tips:

1. Wholesome Help: Menopause is related to hormonal changes that can influence digestion and supplement prerequisites. Embracing a decent and supplement-rich eating regimen can uphold generally speaking well-being during this stage. Counseling an enlisted dietitian can assist with guaranteeing you're getting sufficient supplements while dealing with particular side effects.

2. Liver Help: The liver assumes a fundamental part in chemical digestion and detoxification. Supporting liver well-being through a decent eating routine, ordinary activity, and keeping away from unnecessary liquor utilization can be gainful.

3. Stress The executives: Menopause can achieve physical and profound pressure. Participating in pressure the executives' methods like contemplation, profound breathing activities, or participating in

exercises you appreciate can assist with supporting general prosperity.

4. Standard Activity: Actual work can assist with overseeing weight, support bone wellbeing, further develop temperament, and decrease menopausal side effects. Talk with your medical care supplier to decide the most suitable workout daily practice for you.

5. Satisfactory Rest: Menopause can upset rest designs. Focus on quality rest by keeping a reliable rest plan, establishing a helpful rest climate, and rehearsing great rest cleanliness.

Keep in mind, every individual's involvement in menopause is one of a kind, and what works for one individual may not work for another. It's essential to talk with a medical care proficient who can evaluate your particular necessities and give customized direction and proposals custom-made to your circumstance.

Menopause-explicit treatments or medicines, like chemical substitution treatment (HRT), may likewise be considered for overseeing menopausal side effects. These ought to be examined with a medical care supplier who can gauge the possible advantages and dangers in light of your clinical history and individual conditions.

CHAPTER SEVEN: STAYING YOUNG

Tragically, it isn't as of now feasible for people to remain youthful for eternity. Maturing is a characteristic natural interaction that influences generally living life forms, and keeping in mind that there are different ways of advancing solid maturing and keeping a young appearance, they can't stop the maturing system completely. Be that as it may, there are a few hints on the most proficient method to improve with age and keep up with great well-being:

1. Solid way of life: Taking on a sound way of life can fundamentally influence your general prosperity and dial back the impacts of maturing. This incorporates standard activity, a decent eating regimen wealthy in natural products, vegetables, and entire grains, keeping a solid weight, and abstaining from smoking or unreasonable liquor utilization.

2. Skincare: Dealing with your skin can assist with limiting the noticeable indications of maturing.

Safeguard your skin from the sun by wearing sunscreen and defensive dress, saturate consistently, and use skincare items that suit your skin type.

3. Stress the executives: Persistent pressure can speed up maturing and adversely influence your well-being. Practice pressure-the-board strategies like reflection, profound breathing activities, yoga, or taking part in leisure activities and exercises you appreciate to assist with diminishing feelings of anxiety.

4. Remain intellectually dynamic: Keep your psyche dynamic by taking part in intellectually animating exercises. Understand books, tackle puzzles, master new abilities, or take part in exercises that challenge your mind to keep up with mental capability.

5. Social associations: Keeping up areas of strength for associations and participating in significant connections can add to by and large prosperity and assist with combatting sensations of dejection or disengagement, which can affect your well-being and personal satisfaction.

6. Quality rest: Get adequate and serene rest to help your body's regular revival processes. Lay out a customary rest schedule, establish an agreeable rest climate, and stay away from propensities that can upset rest, for example, over-the-top screen time before bed.

7. Standard well-being check-ups: Visit your medical services supplier routinely for preventive screenings and check-ups. Tending to medical problems proactively can assist with overseeing them actually and advance by and large prosperity.

Keep in mind, maturing is a characteristic piece of life, and embracing the various stages while zeroing in on keeping up with great well-being and an uplifting perspective is fundamental.